Rejuvenate and Restore

Rejuvenate and Restore

The Complete Guide to Postpartum Stretches

Kyann Sharp

For all the women that have been by my side, supporting my journey through motherhood.

Table of Contents

Introduction

Bringing a new life into this world is a remarkable journey, but it can also take a toll on your body. Postpartum recovery is a crucial phase for new mothers, and one of the most effective ways to support your body during this time is through postpartum stretches. In this comprehensive guide, we will explore the importance of postpartum stretching, various stretches tailored to your specific needs, and how to safely integrate them into your postpartum routine.

Chapter 1: The Postpartum Journey

Understanding the postpartum period

After delivery, the next stage in a mother's life is the postpartum period, which is a crucial and challenging time. This is a recovery period after childbirth. This stage is the period of time when the mother's body's numerous organ systems experience thorough healing and restoration. It lasts until the mother's altered physiology and anatomy return to what they were before being pregnant. It can be divided into three related phases.

1. **Acute Phase (0-12 Hours Postpartum):**

This is the stage that immediately follows childbirth. It starts within the first 12 hours of the baby's life. In this stage, the uterus contracts and shrinks back to its pre-pregnancy size as a result of the mother's body starting the process of uterine involution. There are significant hormonal changes, including the decrease in progesterone and the release of oxytocin, which facilitates breastfeeding and bonding between the mother and child.

1. **Subacute Phase (0-6 Weeks Postpartum):**

This period lasts for roughly six weeks and is characterized by a variety of emotional and physical changes. It's characterized by the gradual restoration of the mother's body to its pre-pregnancy state. During this period, the mother may experience significant hormonal fluctuations, mood swings, and physical recovery. Her reproductive organs, as well as other body systems, undergo the process of healing and adaptation.

1. **Delayed Phase (Up to 6 Months Postpartum):**

The delayed phase is a prolonged period of the postpartum journey that can last up to six months. Certain physiological changes, particularly those affecting the genitourinary system, may take a long time to heal during this time. This is especially important in the case of urine incontinence, when the effects of pregnancy and childbirth on the pelvic floor muscles may necessitate additional time for recovery and rehabilitation.

Physical and emotional changes after childbirth

In the initial days and weeks following childbirth, significant hormonal fluctuations occur, giving rise to a range of physical and emotional transformations.

After giving birth, the body experiences an increase in endorphins and oxytocin levels. This results in a strong bond between mother and child, which relieves stress. Also, the removal of the placenta triggers a decrease in estrogen and progesterone levels, which potentially contributes to what is commonly referred to as the "baby blues" or postpartum depression (PPD). The baby blues cause mood swings, episodes of crying, and heightened anxiety, typically resolving on their own within a brief period.

PPD affects a large number of moms, with around one in every eight experiencing symptoms. It emerges as intense feelings of despair, anxiety, or hopelessness that interfere with daily activities and last for weeks after delivery.

Also, regardless of whether you had a vaginal or C-section delivery, you may have physical discomfort during your postpartum recovery. Sleep deprivation increases the challenges that you face as a mother.

It's important to recognize that hormonal fluctuations, combined with external stressors like sleep deprivation and pain, can strongly influence your mental well-being. With the right support and as your body undergoes the healing process, most individuals notice an improvement in their condition after a few weeks. Remember to be patient with yourself as the healing journey unfolds.

The role of stretching in postpartum recovery

Stretching is highly important in postpartum recovery since it provides new mothers with a gentle and effective way to renew their bodies and increase their well-being. The physical toll of childbirth, with stretching and contraction of muscles, often leaves mothers in need of healing and restoration.

Stretching after giving birth can help with this process by reducing muscle tension, which improves flexibility and encourages improved blood circulation. These simple body movements address the unique needs of postpartum bodies, reducing discomfort. They also foster an important bond between a mother and her body, allowing her to regain strength and confidence as she begins the beautiful yet challenging task of parenting.

Postpartum stretches also provide a sanctuary for emotional healing. They offer a precious moment of self-care amid the whirlwind of caring for a newborn, which allows mothers to reconnect with themselves. As they stretch and breathe, mothers whisper promises of love, healing, and gratitude to their bodies, acknowledging the incredible journey they have shared. In this nurturing practice, mothers find not only physical relief but also emotional resilience. The postpartum period is a time of great transformation, and stretching is a very important tool that gently guides mothers toward recovery, self-acceptance, and the celebration of their remarkable strength.

Chapter 2: Preparing for Postpartum Stretches

Safety considerations

Safety is paramount when preparing for postpartum stretches. As a new mother, you should pay careful attention to the following considerations to ensure a safe and effective postpartum stretching routine.

- **Consult with a Healthcare Professional:** Before beginning any postpartum exercise, including stretching, it's important to consult with your healthcare provider. They can assess your individual health, any complications from childbirth, and provide suitable advice based on your specific needs.

- **Listen to Your Body:** You should pay close attention to your body's signals. If you experience pain or discomfort during a stretch, stop immediately. Your body is still recovering, and it's essential to respect its limits.

- **Start Gradually:** Make sure that you begin with gentle and simple stretches. Postpartum bodies are more susceptible to injury, so gradual progression is key. Over time, you can increase the intensity and duration of your stretches.

- **Avoid Overstretching:** Hormonal changes during pregnancy can lead to increased joint flexibility, so be cautious not to overstretch. Use controlled, mindful movements rather than forceful stretching.

- **Stay Hydrated:** Proper hydration is important for general health and muscle performance. Drinking enough water helps prevent muscle cramps and supports tissue repair.

- **Breathing and Relaxation:** Incorporate deep, mindful breathing during your stretches. This not only enhances relaxation but also helps in maintaining proper form and reducing tension.

- **Posture and Alignment:** Focus on maintaining good posture and alignment during your stretches to prevent strain on your muscles and joints.

- **Supportive Environment:** Create a safe, clutter-free space for your stretching routine. Ensure the surface is comfortable, and use a mat or blanket for added cushioning.

- **Watch for Signs of Diastasis Recti:** Diastasis recti is a pregnancy problem in which the abdominal muscles separate. If you suspect you have this condition, consult with a physical therapist to learn safe abdominal exercises and avoid exacerbating the separation.

- **Include Warm-Up and Cool-Down:** Always start with a brief warm-up to prepare your muscles and finish with a cool-down to help prevent stiffness.

Setting up a postpartum stretching routine

To ensure that your stretching routine complements your postpartum self-care and doesn't become an additional source of stress, here's a more detailed approach.

Prioritize Basic Self-Care:

Your initial focus in the early postpartum phase should be on self-care, alongside caring for your newborn. Ensure you're eating nutritious meals daily to support your physical recovery and provide the energy needed to care for your baby. Stay well-hydrated with plenty of water, and whenever possible, try to get adequate rest. Personal hygiene and recovery from pregnancy and childbirth are also fundamental aspects of your self-care during this period.

Keep Stretching Goals Realistic:

Understand that your body is still in a state of healing and adjustment. Your stretching routine should enhance your well-being rather than add to your stress. Therefore, set achievable goals and don't pressure yourself to perform complex stretches or follow an intensive routine immediately. Start with gentle, basic stretches to promote flexibility and relaxation.

Balance To-Do Lists:

While you might have home or work-related tasks you'd like to complete, it's crucial not to overwhelm yourself. Limit your daily to-do list to just a couple of manageable tasks. This approach prevents feelings of being overwhelmed and disappointed if you cannot accomplish an extensive list. By focusing on only two tasks a day, you can achieve small wins and gradually build your self-confidence over time.

Incorporate Stretching into Your Routine:

Integrate your postpartum stretching routine into your daily schedule in a way that feels natural and manageable. For example, you might choose to stretch during your baby's naptime or as a brief relaxation break during the day. This way, it becomes part of your daily self-care, alongside other essential activities.

Be Patient with Yourself:

Recognize that postpartum recovery is a unique journey for every individual. It's perfectly acceptable to adapt and modify your stretching routine as your body and energy levels change. If you have days when you can do more, that's great. If you have days when you can only manage a short, gentle stretch, that's perfectly fine as well.

By striking this balance between postpartum stretching and self-care, you can ensure that your stretching routine remains a supportive and positive addition to your postpartum life, aiding in your physical and emotional recovery without overwhelming you with unrealistic expectations. Remember that self-compassion and flexibility are key as you go through this period.

Consultation with healthcare professionals

In order to ensure that new mothers have a safe and successful recovery process, consulting with healthcare professionals about postpartum stretches is essential. Healthcare professionals, including obstetricians, physical therapists, or certified postpartum fitness instructors, possess valuable expertise that can be tailored to an individual's specific postpartum needs. They offer insights into the unique physical changes and challenges associated with pregnancy and childbirth, helping mothers understand the limitations and precautions required during the postpartum period.

Healthcare professionals can assess the mother's overall health and any complications from childbirth, making personalized recommendations and advising on when it's appropriate to initiate a stretching routine. This guidance ensures that the chosen stretches align with the mother's current health status and will not hinder the recovery process.

Also, healthcare professionals can suggest specialized stretches that target specific postpartum concerns, such as pelvic floor issues or abdominal muscle separation. Furthermore, they provide essential advice on posture, form, and gradual progression to prevent injuries. Their knowledge assists moms in navigating the often complicated postpartum setting, which leads to a safe, supportive, and ultimately successful stretching routine that adds to the physical and mental well-being of new mothers during this transforming stage of life.

Consulting healthcare professionals is a proactive and responsible approach to postpartum stretching, ensuring that mothers receive the best guidance and care to facilitate a smooth and healthful recovery.

Chapter 3: Gentle Stretches for Early Postpartum

Gentle stretching is an excellent way to ease into postpartum recovery, promoting both physical well-being and relaxation. Here are some specific stretches that can be particularly beneficial during the early postpartum period.

Neck and shoulder stretches

Neck and shoulder stretches are beneficial for relieving tension and discomfort in the upper body, which is particularly common during the postpartum period when new mothers often spend extended periods cradling their babies. Here are some simple neck and shoulder stretches to try.

Neck Tilts:

To perform this stretch, sit or stand with your back straight in a comfortable position. Next, turn your head slightly to the side and bring your ear close to your shoulder. Feel the mild strain along the side of your neck as you hold the pose for 15 to 30 seconds. Repeat on the opposite side. This stretch aids in releasing muscle tension in the neck.

Neck Rolls:

Start from the same sitting or standing position, maintaining a straight back. Bring your ear toward your shoulder by rolling your head to one side after lowering your chin gradually to your chest. Keep rotating your head to the opposite side and return to the initial position. The stress in the shoulders and neck can be relieved with these slow, gentle neck rolls.

Shoulder Rolls:

Place your arms down by your sides and your feet hip-width apart. For 10 to 15 seconds, move your shoulders forward in a circular motion. Next, turn the other way around and roll your shoulders back. For releasing shoulder strain and enhancing posture, try this stretch.

Shoulder Blade Squeeze:

Maintain a straight back whether you are sitting or standing. Squeeze your shoulder blades together gently. Hold for a short while, then let go. The rounded shoulder position that can result from nursing and holding a newborn is countered by this stretch.

Upper Trapezius Stretch:

With your feet flat on the ground, take a seat in a chair. With one hand, grasp the bottom of the chair, and then slowly tilt your head to the other side, bringing your ear closer to your shoulder. By using your palm to gently apply pressure, you can enhance the stretch. Switch to the other side after holding for 15 to 30 seconds.

You should regularly stretch your neck and shoulders, especially when you're taking little breaks from caring for your child. They can make your postpartum experience more comfortable and joyful by easing tense muscles and enhancing your general comfort. If you feel pain or discomfort when performing these stretches, seek advice from a healthcare provider.

Ankle and foot stretches

Ankle and foot stretches are excellent for alleviating discomfort, particularly when postpartum swelling, fluid retention, and changes in posture can affect the lower extremities. Here are some simple ankle and foot stretches to consider.

Toe Flex and Point:

Sit down comfortably with your legs extended. Start by flexing your toes toward your shins, feeling a gentle stretch in the calf muscles. Hold for a few seconds, and then point your toes away from your body, stretching the tops of your feet. Alternate between flexing and pointing for a minute or two to improve circulation and reduce foot swelling.

Ankle Circles:

While seated or lying down, lift one foot slightly off the ground. Rotate your ankle in a clockwise motion, making slow circles. After a few rotations, reverse the direction and circle counterclockwise.

This stretch helps maintain ankle flexibility and reduce ankle stiffness.

Towel Stretch:

Place a towel beneath the arch of one of your feet and sit with your legs outstretched. Hold both ends of the towel with your hands and gently draw the towel toward you while keeping your leg straight. This stretch relieves the arch of the foot and the calf.

Foot Flex and Point:

Sit with your legs extended. Point your toes away from your body and then flex them toward your shins. This stretch helps relieve tension in the calf and the sole of the foot. Repeat the motion for a minute or two on each foot.

Achilles Stretch:

Place your hands against the wall as you stand facing it. Bend your front knee and take a single step back, keeping your foot flat on the ground. To feel a stretch along the Achilles tendon and calf of the back leg, slant your hips forward. After holding for 15 to 30 seconds, move your weight to the other foot.

Regularly performing these ankle and foot stretches can help reduce swelling, increase circulation, and relieve tension in the lower extremities, all of which can be particularly comforting during the postpartum period. If you experience discomfort or have specific foot-related concerns, consult with a healthcare provider or a physical therapist for personalized guidance.

Pelvic floor exercises

Pelvic floor exercises are very important during the postpartum recovery process, especially after vaginal childbirth. These exercises strengthen the pelvic floor muscles. Though you can use your pelvic floor muscles anywhere and at any time, it can be useful to know which exercises are best for your hypotonic and hypertonic pelvic floor muscles in order to treat specific issues in a systematic manner.

Hypotonic Exercises

Quick Flick Kegels:

Begin lying down with knees bent and feet flat. Contract and release your pelvic floor muscles quickly while exhaling, aiming for a one-second contraction. Maintain steady breathing and complete 10 repetitions per set. Rest for 10 seconds between sets. This exercise enhances muscle strength and responsiveness, particularly helpful in preventing leaks during activities like sneezing or coughing.

Heel Slides:

Lie with knees bent and a neutral pelvis position. Inhale, then exhale while drawing your pelvic floor up, engaging your deep core. Slide one heel away from your body while maintaining core engagement. Inhale and return to the starting position. Repeat for

10 repetitions with each leg. This exercise promotes pelvic floor contractions and deep abdominal muscle engagement, enhancing core stability.

Marches (Toe Taps):

Similar to heel slides, this exercise encourages pelvic floor contractions and core stability. Lie with knees bent and a neutral pelvis. Inhale, then exhale while lifting one leg to a tabletop position, ensuring your deep core remains contracted. For about 12–20 repetitions, slowly lower the leg to the starting position while switching between legs.

Hypertonic Exercises

Happy Baby Pose:

This stretch focuses on relaxation and lengthening, making it valuable for individuals with hypertonic pelvic floor muscles. Begin by lying down with knees bent. Pull your knees toward your belly at a 90-degree angle, holding the outside or inside of your feet. Your feet should be close to your armpits as you open your knees wider than your chest. Flex your heels and gently rock from side to side, providing a release for tight pelvic floor muscles.

Diaphragmatic Breathing:

This exercise promotes the functional relationship between the diaphragm and the pelvic floor. It encourages relaxation and may reduce stress. Start by sitting or lying flat on the ground. After gradually relaxing for a few seconds, pay attention to your breathing. Inhale through your nose, expanding your stomach while keeping your chest still. Exhale slowly, repeating several times with one hand on your chest and the other on your stomach.

Modified Plank:

Begin in a tabletop position on your hands and knees, then extend one leg behind you with your foot on the ground. Lift this extended leg while engaging your pelvic floor, and subsequently lower it before switching to the other leg.

Pelvic floor exercises are effective in preventing or alleviating issues such as urinary incontinence and pelvic organ prolapse, as well as enhancing postpartum recovery. They can also help with sexual function and sensation. These exercises are beneficial not only for postpartum recovery but also for long-term pelvic health.

Chapter 4: Core Restoration

Diastasis recti

Diastasis recti refers to the separation of the rectus abdominis muscles both during and following gestation. It is a common issue. The rectus abdominis, often known as the "six-pack," runs vertically in the front of the abdomen, divided into left and right sides by the linea alba. The expanding uterus stretches the abdominal muscles, which causes the linea alba to thin and widen, during pregnancy. After childbirth, the linea alba can naturally heal because of its elastic properties. However, if it loses elasticity due to excessive stretching, it may not close as it should, leading to diastasis recti. This condition results in a noticeable protrusion above or below the belly button, often lasting long after giving birth.

How to address diastasis recti

To address diastasis recti, engage in gentle abdominal muscle movements after ensuring their safety with a professional experienced in diastasis recti. Collaborate with a fitness expert or physical therapist to develop a suitable treatment plan, ensuring proper execution of exercises and gradual progression to more challenging routines.

During the postpartum phase, exercise caution with certain activities:

- Avoid lifting items heavier than your baby.

- Safely rise from a supine position by rolling onto your side and using your arms for support.

- Exclude exercises that exert outward pressure on your abdominal muscles, such as crunches and sit-ups.

While some individuals use binding devices, like elastic belly bands, to provide temporary support, these do not heal diastasis recti or strengthen your core muscles. However, they can serve as a helpful reminder of your condition and promote better posture.

Abdominal stretches

Prior to starting abdominal exercises, consult your healthcare provider to prevent injury during postpartum recovery, especially after a C-section. C-sections require more recovery time than vaginal births. Strengthen your core comprehensively, focusing on stabilizer muscles, for improved connective tissue and range of motion. These post-pregnancy workouts are a great way to revitalize your postpartum belly. Start with 1-2 short sets of 10 reps, increasing gradually to 3-4 sets as your strength improves.

Pelvic Bridge

The pelvic bridge and deep belly breathing are familiar yoga exercises. The bridge (setu bandha sarvangasana) is a foundational backbend yoga pose that strengthens the lower back and hip muscles, and lengthens the abs. Here's how to activate the targeted muscles:

1. Rest on your back, legs bent, and place your feet flat on the mat.

2. Maintaining your head, neck, and shoulders on the floor, raise your pelvis.

3. Draw your knees together if you can, instead of spreading them apart.

4. After three breaths of holding, slowly lower yourself and repeat.

Bridge pose lengthens and strengthens spine-supporting muscles, making it a great morning energizer.

Horizontal Forearm Plank

This exercise effectively builds full-body strength, particularly targeting the upper back and shoulders, making it an ideal body-weight exercise. Don't be discouraged by its initial challenge; it has modifications to gradually progress.

1. Start in a tabletop position.

2. Shift to parallel forearms for stability.

3. Extend knees to create a straight line from neck to knees.

4. Engage core and pelvic floor, and hold for 30 seconds.

5. Then try it off your knees for three breaths.

6. Once comfortable, aim for a one-minute hold.

Diastasis recti patients should seek a specialized physiotherapist for personalized exercises.

Side Plank

The side plank is a potent full-body exercise that complements the forearm plank, targeting obliques and shoulders. To execute:

1. Begin by lying on your side, legs fully extended, and your forearm supporting your upper body (ensure your shoulder aligns with your elbow).

2. Elevate your hips until your body forms a straight line from shoulders to ankles.

3. Envision being between two glass panes, preventing shoulder hunching and expanding through your chest.

4. If strong, lift one leg toward the ceiling.

5. Maintain the side plank for 30 seconds.

6. The next level is transitioning from your forearm to balancing on your hand.

7. Balance can be challenging; focus your gaze on a stationary object and maintain steady breathing.

Bent Leg Raises

Bent leg raises should be initiated with your doctor's approval due to the potential intensity they bring to your lower abdominals and hip flexors. These muscles play a crucial role in relieving lower back pain, which often arises when they lack sufficient strength.

You might begin with the straight leg raise version to get yourself ready for the full activity and lower your chance of injury. To perform this exercise:

1. Begin by lying on a mat, arms by your sides, knees bent, and feet flat on the floor.

2. Once you feel ready to advance, try raising and lowering both legs simultaneously.

3. Alternate legs deliberately, focusing on controlled movements to engage the stabilizing muscles.

4. Engage your core, drawing your belly button toward your spine, and raise one leg toward your chest before returning it to the starting position.

Progressing in this manner will help you develop the strength needed for straight-leg raises, transforming this into a formidable ab workout.

Deep Belly Breathing

This exercise focuses on the diaphragm, positioned at the chest's base, primarily responsible for expanding the chest cavity during breathing. It collaborates with abdominal muscles and the pelvic floor to stabilize the body's trunk. Here's how to do it:

1. Lie on your back, knees bent, feet flat on a yoga mat or towel.

2. Fill your lungs by inhaling softly through your nose.

3. Place one hand on your chest and one on your belly button to sense chest and belly expansion.

4. Exhale with control through your mouth, feeling your stomach and chest moving closer to your spine as you release the air.

5. Begin with four-count inhales, pausing at the breath's peak, and exhale in four counts, gradually increasing breath length with practice.

This exercise is gentle postpartum and offers numerous health benefits, including stress reduction, improved lung capacity, strengthened abdominal and pelvic floor muscles, reduced heart rate, and lower blood pressure.

Strengthening the pelvic floor muscles

Pelvic floor exercises work on the muscles that surround the bladder, pelvis, and genital area. These exercises help with urinary tract problems, pelvic organ prolapse, and sexual satisfaction. To perform these exercises:

1. Sit comfortably and perform 10-15 muscle contractions without holding your breath or engaging other muscle groups.

2. As you advance, try to hold each contraction for a few seconds.

3. Increase repetitions gradually each week, with appropriate rest between sets to avoid overexertion.

Improvements are visible after a few months. Consistency is key; continue the exercises even as benefits become noticeable. Some of these exercises are as follows:

Kegel Exercises: Involve contracting the muscles around your vaginal and anal area, as if halting urination, holding for a few seconds before releasing and repeating.

Bridge Pose: Lie on your back with knees bent and feet flat, raising your hips off the ground to activate your pelvic floor, then lower.

Squats: Stand with feet hip-width apart, lower into a squat with a straight back, and engage your pelvic floor when rising.

Wall Squats: These are similar to squats but performed against a wall, sliding down while bending your knees and pushing back up, engaging the pelvic floor.

Chapter 5: Relieving Back and Hip Pain

Back and hip pain can be incredibly debilitating, affecting not only our physical well-being but also our overall quality of life. Whether you're dealing with chronic discomfort, recovering from pregnancy, or simply looking to improve flexibility and strength in these areas, there are various stretches and exercises that can help alleviate these issues.

Stretches to Alleviate Back Pain

Child's Pose:

This classic yoga pose can help with lower back pain alleviation by gently stretching the lower back. Kneel on the floor with your big toes touching and knees apart. Lower your chest toward the floor while sitting back on your heels and extending your arms forward on the floor. Hold this stretch for 20-30 seconds, breathing deeply.

Cat-Cow Stretch:

This stretch is a dynamic movement that increases spinal flexibility and relieves back tension. Begin in a tabletop position, arch your back, lift your head and tailbone (Cow Pose) while inhaling, and then exhale as you round your back and tuck your chin (Cat Pose). Repeat this stretch 10-15 times.

Knee-to-Chest Stretch:

While lying on your back, gently draw one knee toward your chest, using both hands to support the movement. Keep your opposite leg fully extended. Maintain this position for a duration of 20 to 30 seconds before transitioning to the other leg. This stretching exercise can be beneficial in alleviating tension in the hips and lower back.

Hip-Opening Stretches

Pigeon Pose:

The pigeon pose serves as an effective method for opening up the hips. Start the pose from a plank position, bringing one knee forward to the outer edge of your mat, while the other leg remains fully extended behind you. Gradually ease into the stretch, ensuring that your hips remain in a square position. Maintain the posture for a duration of 30 seconds on both sides.

Butterfly Stretch:

Get in a seated position on the ground with the soles of your feet in contact. Hold your feet using your hands and apply gentle pressure to lower your knees toward the floor. This stretching exercise is designed to focus on the inner thighs and hip flexors.

Lizard Pose:

From a plank position, step one foot forward to the outside of your hand. Lower your hips and forearms to the ground. This intense stretch opens the hips and can provide relief to hip discomfort.

Yoga for Postpartum Recovery

Modified Bridge Pose:

Lie on your back with your knees bent and feet flat on the floor. Lift your hips off the ground, engaging your glutes and core. This helps strengthen the pelvic floor and lower back, which is particularly beneficial for postpartum recovery.

Cobbler's Pose:

Gently bend your knees and allow them to fall outward as you bring the soles of your feet together, drawing them in toward your body within your comfort range, being cautious to prevent knee discomfort. Engage the outer edges of your feet to promote a book-like opening, using your hands or adopting a yogi toe lock by gripping your big toes. Maintain an upright posture with an elongated spine, ensuring your shoulder blades are retracted and your shoulders are relaxed away from your ears.

Savasana (Corpse Pose):

End your postpartum yoga routine with this relaxation pose. Lie on your back, close your eyes, and focus on deep breathing. It helps reduce stress, promotes relaxation, and is essential for overall well-being.

Relieving back and hip discomfort involves a blend of stretches, hip-opening routines, and postpartum yoga, which can notably enhance your well-being. Consistent practice is crucial, along with consulting a healthcare professional or certified yoga instructor, particularly if you have pre-existing health issues.

Chapter 6: Reconnecting with Your Body

In our fast-paced digital age, it's easy to disconnect from our bodies due to daily pressures, constant notifications, and rapid modern living. This disconnection can lead to increased stress, anxiety, and reduced well-being. To address this, reconnecting through mindfulness, relaxation, deep breathing, and progressive muscle relaxation is a powerful solution.

Mindfulness and Relaxation Techniques

Mindfulness is a technique that leads to a strong feeling of being alive, emphasizing the observation of thoughts, emotions, and sensations without making judgments. By directing your focus toward your body, you can initiate the process of reconnection. Here are some beneficial mindfulness and relaxation methods to aid in this endeavor.

Body Scan Meditation:

This meditation involves a systematic focus on each part of your body. Start from your toes and work your way up to your head, paying attention to any tension, discomfort, or sensations you feel in each area. As you go through this process, you'll become more aware of how your body feels, and this heightened awareness can foster a deeper connection.

Yoga:

Yoga combines physical postures with mindfulness and deep breathing. The practice of yoga encourages the alignment of body and mind, making it an excellent way to reconnect with your body. Through various poses and stretches, you can explore your body's abilities and limitations, while also enhancing flexibility and strength.

Progressive Muscle Relaxation (PMR):

The PMR technique involves tensing and relaxing particular muscle groups. This process helps you identify and release tension in your body. As you systematically move through different muscle groups, you become acutely aware of the sensations in each area. This awareness helps you release pent-up stress and tension.

Mindful Eating:

Paying close attention to the sensory experiences of eating can be a great way to reconnect with your body. Enjoy every bite of your food by taking time to appreciate its flavors, textures, and even sounds. Mindful eating can help you appreciate the nourishment your body receives and recognize feelings of hunger and fullness more effectively.

Breathing Exercises

Breathing is a fundamental bodily function, yet we often take it for granted. Learning to breathe consciously and intentionally can significantly aid in reconnecting with your body and calming your mind. Here are some breathing exercises that can help.

Deep Belly Breathing:

Find a comfortable sitting or lying position, with one hand on your chest and the other on your belly. Inhale deeply through your nose, expanding your diaphragm, causing your abdomen to rise. Exhale slowly through your mouth, noting the descent of your chest and belly. This deep belly breathing promotes nervous system relaxation and enhances your bodily grounding.

4-7-8 Breathing:

This technique lowers stress and encourages relaxation. Quietly breathe in through your nose for four counts, hold for seven, and exhale through your mouth for eight counts. Repeat this process for a few cycles, and you'll notice a sense of calm and reconnection with your body.

Box Breathing:

Box breathing is a simple and effective method for recentering yourself. Breathe in for four counts, hold it for four, release it for four counts, then repeat the process for a total of four counts. This creates a square pattern, helping you stay focused and present in your body.

Progressive Muscle Relaxation

Progressive Muscle Relaxation (PMR), as previously discussed, is a potent method for reestablishing a connection with your body. It involves tensing and subsequently releasing various muscle groups to alleviate physical tension and stress. Here's how to implement it:

1. Find a quiet, comfortable space where you won't be disturbed.

2. Start with your toes and work your way up through your body. For each muscle group, tense the muscles for 5-10 seconds, and then release.

3. Focus on the sensations as you release the tension. Notice the contrast between tension and relaxation.

4. Continue moving up your body, including your legs, abdomen, chest, arms, and face.

5. As you complete each muscle group, take a moment to enjoy the deep sense of relaxation.

Progressive Muscle Relaxation can be especially helpful in identifying and releasing bodily tension. It allows you to cultivate a greater sense of physical awareness and control.

In conclusion, reconnecting with your body through mindfulness, relaxation exercises, and breath work is crucial in today's fast-paced, tech-centric world. These practices reduce stress and anxiety while enhancing your presence in your own body, promoting overall well-being and balance.

Chapter 7: Postpartum Stretches for Different Delivery Methods

During this time, mothers often experience discomfort, muscle tightness, and a need for recovery, depending on the method of childbirth they underwent. Whether a vaginal birth, a cesarean section (C-section), or the birth of multiples, each delivery method presents unique considerations for postpartum recovery.

Stretching for Vaginal Birth

Vaginal birth is the typical childbirth method, frequently leading to perineal stretching and potential tearing. These stretches can help ease discomfort and facilitate recovery.

Kegel Exercises:

Kegel exercises are a crucial component of postpartum recovery for vaginal births. These exercises target the pelvic floor muscles, helping to strengthen and tone them. To do a Kegel exercise, contract and release the same muscles as if you were stopping the flow of urine. Hold for a few seconds, release, and repeat multiple times daily.

Pelvic Tilts:

Pelvic tilts enhance lower back and abdominal muscle flexibility and strength. To boost abdominal strength, lie on your back with knees bent, engage your ab muscles to flatten your back against the floor, and gently lift your pelvis, holding for up to 10 seconds before repeating.

Deep Squats:

Deep squats relax and elongate pelvic floor muscles and stretch the perineum. Start by standing with legs wider than hip width, squatting as low as possible with hands together in front of you. Consult your physical therapist for guidance on the frequency and quantity of deep squats recommended.

Butterfly Stretch:

The butterfly stretch targets the inner thighs and groin muscles, which can be tight after a vaginal birth. Sit on the floor with the soles of your feet together and your knees bent outward. Gently press your knees toward the floor, feeling a stretch in your inner thighs. Hold for 20-30 seconds, and repeat a few times.

Cat-Cow Stretch:

This yoga-inspired stretch helps alleviate back pain and improves posture. Get on your hands and knees, then inhale and exhale while arching your back upward (Cat Pose) and downward (Cow Pose). Repeat this movement many times to relieve back strain.

Child's Pose:

This yoga pose is excellent for relaxation and stretching. Assume a kneeling position with your toes touching and your knees spaced apart. Gently lower your body onto your heels and extend your arms forward, resting them on the floor. Maintain this posture for as long as it remains comfortable.

Stretching for Cesarean Section Recovery

Cesarean section deliveries involve an incision in the abdominal wall, which requires specialized postpartum care. Here are some gentle stretches that can aid in C-section recovery.

Deep Breathing and Abdominal Contraction:

Begin by inhaling deeply to increase the oxygen supply to your abdominal muscles. During the exhalation, softly contract your abdominal muscles in a manner similar to performing a Kegel exercise. This approach helps in revitalizing core strength without placing undue stress on the surgical site.

Ankle Pumps:

After a C-section, it's important to avoid straining your abdominal muscles. Ankle pumps help improve circulation and prevent blood clots without engaging the core. While lying on your back, flex and point your feet, repeating the motion for a few minutes.

Seated Leg Lifts:

Take a seat on a chair or bed, ensuring your posture is upright. Slowly raise one leg, maintaining its extension, before gently lowering it. Perform the same action with the opposite leg. This workout aids in fortifying your leg muscles while minimizing strain on your surgical incision.

Shoulder Blade Squeezes:

This routine is designed to focus on the upper back and shoulder muscles, which may experience tension when tending to your infant. Whether you choose to sit or stand, begin with your arms resting at your sides. Proceed by gently contracting your shoulder blades toward each other, maintaining this position for a brief moment before relaxing.

Gentle Standing Side Stretch:

Begin by positioning your feet at a distance equivalent to the width of your hips and interlock your hands above your head. Slowly incline your body to one side, experiencing a stretching sensation along your midsection. Return to the starting position, and then replicate the same movement on the opposite side.

Stretches for Mothers of Multiples

Mothers who give birth to multiples, such as twins or triplets, often have unique postpartum challenges. They may experience more significant muscle strain and fatigue. Here are some stretches tailored to their needs.

Legs-Up-the-Wall Pose:

Practicing this calming yoga posture can provide relief for swollen feet and legs. Begin by sitting with your hip positioned next to a wall. Afterward, gently elevate your legs against the wall and recline, extending your arms outward. Take a few minutes in this relaxed position.

Modified Cat-Cow Stretch:

As mentioned before, the cat-cow stretch can help alleviate back pain. For mothers of multiples, this stretch can be modified while sitting on a stability ball to reduce pressure on the lower back and engage the core.

Supported Bridge Pose:

Lie on your back with your knees bent and your feet flat on the floor. Place a cushion or yoga block under your hips and lift your hips off the ground. This stretch helps strengthen the glutes and relieve lower back pain.

Hip Flexor Stretch:

Position yourself on the ground with one knee flexed at a 90-degree angle while extending the other leg to the rear. Gently move your hips forward until you feel your hip flexor muscles stretching. Stay in this posture for 20-30 seconds before switching to the other side.

Pec Stretch:

To ease tension for mothers caring for multiple babies and frequently carrying and feeding them, try this chest stretch. Stand in a doorway with arms extended along the door frame and gently lean forward.

Prior to starting any postpartum exercise or stretching regimen, particularly if you're a mother of multiples or have undergone a C-section, it's crucial to seek guidance from a healthcare expert. They can offer tailored recommendations and guarantee your well-being throughout the recovery journey.

The postpartum period can be both challenging and rewarding for mothers, regardless of the delivery method. The right stretches and exercises can aid in the recovery process, promote physical well-being, and provide some much-needed relaxation during this transformative time. Whether you've had a vaginal birth, a C-section, or are the proud mother of multiples, these stretches can help you regain strength, flexibility, and overall health, allowing you to focus on what truly matters: your new family.

Chapter 8: Incorporating Stretches into Daily Life

Balancing motherhood and self-care

Balancing motherhood and self-care is a delicate juggling act that many mothers face daily. While the demands of caring for children are fulfilling, they can also be overwhelming, often leaving mothers with little time or energy to prioritize self-care. However, it's crucial for mothers to find a balance that ensures their well-being while nurturing their families.

Self-care is not selfish; it's a necessary component of effective motherhood. It involves allocating time for activities that rejuvenate the mind and body, such as exercise, meditation, or pursuing personal interests. These moments of self-indulgence can help reduce stress, boost self-esteem, and promote overall happiness.

To strike this balance, mothers can establish routines that allow for regular self-care intervals, even if they are brief. Support from partners, family members, or friends can be invaluable in providing opportunities for mothers to recharge. Additionally, seeking childcare assistance or organizing playdates can free up moments for self-care.

Ultimately, a well-balanced mother can provide better care to her children. By recognizing that self-care is not only permissible but essential, mothers can ensure that they remain healthy, resilient, and more capable of nurturing their families effectively. It's a delicate dance that yields benefits for both mother and child.

Creating a Postpartum Stretching Schedule

Now that we've established the benefits of stretching for mothers, it's time to create a postpartum stretching schedule tailored to your needs. Here's a step-by-step guide to help you get started.

- **Set Realistic Goals**: Begin by setting achievable goals. Whether it's improving flexibility, reducing muscle tension, or increasing your overall well-being, having clear objectives will help you stay motivated.

- **Choose a Convenient Time**: Identify a suitable moment that aligns with your everyday schedule. This could be when your child is napping or engaging in solitary play. Maintaining a regular schedule is essential, so endeavor to adhere to your selected time frame as faithfully as you can.

- **Select a Comfortable Space**: Designate a comfortable area for your stretching routine. It could be your living room, a quiet corner, or even your backyard. Make sure it's a space where you can relax and focus on your stretches without distractions.

- **Start Slowly**: If you're new to stretching, start with simple and gentle stretches. Focus on major muscle groups, like your neck, shoulders, back, and legs. As you become more comfortable, you can gradually incorporate more advanced stretches.

- **Stay Hydrated**: Proper hydration is essential when incorporating stretches into your daily life. Drink plenty of water before and after your stretching routine to keep your muscles well-hydrated and to aid in the recovery process.

- **Listen to Your Body**: Pay close attention to how your body responds during stretches. Never push yourself to the point of pain or discomfort. Stretching should feel like a gentle, controlled release of tension, not a painful endeavor.

- **Seek Professional Guidance**: If you encounter any worries or particular postpartum challenges, it's advisable to seek guidance from a physical therapist or a specialist in postpartum fitness. They can assist you in developing a stretching regimen that is both safe and tailored to your individual situation.

- **Keep a Stretching Journal:** Use a journal to track your routine, noting your feelings before and after each session, any enhancements in flexibility, and changes in your overall well-being.

Making Stretches a Family Affair

Incorporating stretches into your daily life doesn't have to be a solitary endeavor. You can involve your family, including your children and partner, in this healthy habit. Here are some creative ways to make stretching a family affair.

- **Family Stretching Sessions**: Designate a specific time each day for a family stretching session. Gather in a comfortable space and encourage everyone to participate. This is a fantastic way to bond and set a positive example for your children.

- **Playful Stretching**: For younger children, turn stretching into a game. Incorporate imaginative storytelling while stretching or make it a challenge to touch toes, reach for the sky, or mimic animal poses. This approach makes stretching fun and engaging for kids.

- **Partner Stretching**: If your partner is willing, engage in partner stretching sessions. This can be a great way to connect, relieve tension, and encourage mutual self-care.

- **Outdoor Stretching**: Take advantage of the great outdoors by having family stretching sessions in your backyard, at the park, or by the beach. The fresh air and change of scenery can enhance the experience.

- **Dance Breaks**: Put on your favorite music and have spontaneous dance breaks with your children. Dancing is a fantastic way to incorporate stretching and movement into your daily life while enjoying quality time with your family.

Integrating daily stretches can transform your motherhood routine, providing physical and mental advantages, improving well-being, and fostering family connections. Setting achievable goals, adhering to a postpartum stretching regimen, and involving loved ones can help you strike a balance between motherhood and self-care, leading to a healthier and happier you.

Chapter 9: Nutrition and Postpartum Recovery

The role of nutrition in healing

Many physiological changes occur during and after childbirth. The nine-month process of pregnancy results in various bodily adaptations, which take time to revert. Postpartum, your skin regains elasticity, connective tissue repairs, and breast milk production, a metabolically demanding process, begins. Vaginal and C-section deliveries can cause skin tearing and alterations, necessitating specific nutrient support during the healing process. Extended deliveries often lead to calorie expenditure without proper nutrition.

Proper nutrition is essential for several reasons.

Tissue Repair:

Childbirth can lead to tears, incisions, and episiotomies, and it's crucial to ensure sufficient protein intake for proper tissue repair and regeneration. Protein-rich foods like lean meats, fish, legumes, and dairy speed up healing.

Energy Recovery:

Childbirth is physically demanding, and the body needs extra energy for recovery. Complex carbohydrates, in whole grains, fruits, and veggies, offer the energy and fiber for digestive health.

Hormone Regulation:

Postpartum hormonal shifts are common and can lead to mood swings. Foods like fatty fish, flaxseed, and walnuts can stabilize the mood and lower the risk of postpartum depression.

Bone Health:

Pregnancy and breastfeeding can deplete a woman's calcium stores, impacting her bone health. Dairy and leafy greens are vital for preventing issues like osteoporosis.

Breastfeeding Support:

Breastfeeding moms need extra calories and nutrients for quality milk production. A well-balanced diet with ample vitamins and minerals is essential for the well-being of both mother and baby.

Key nutrients for postpartum recovery:

- Calcium is essential due to increased demand during lactation and reduced estrogen levels, impacting bone health.

- Protein aids muscle build, repair, and maintenance, particularly after a C-section.

- Fiber promotes bowel regularity, which can be disrupted by postpartum hormone shifts.

- Hydration is vital for recovery and essential for breastfeeding to support milk production.

- Vitamins and minerals support blood, skin, mood, and lactation health.

Foods to support postpartum recovery

Lean Proteins:

Integrate sources of lean protein, such as chicken, turkey, fish, tofu, and legumes, into your daily nutrition. Protein plays a crucial role in repairing tissues and aiding muscle recuperation. Also, it contributes to stabilizing blood sugar levels, which can have a positive impact on both mood and energy regulation.

Whole Grains:

Choose whole grains for lasting energy and digestive system support, such as brown rice, quinoa, and whole wheat bread.

Fruits and Vegetables:

A variety mix of fruits and veggies provides a wealth of vitamins, minerals, and antioxidants, enhancing the immune system and aiding recovery, with a focus on berries, leafy greens, and citrus fruits.

Healthy Fats:

Incorporate mood-stabilizing foods like avocados, nuts, and olive oil into your diet for emotional balance. These foods are rich in healthy fats.

Dairy Products:

If you're not lactose intolerant, dairy products like yogurt and milk can be excellent sources of calcium. Calcium is crucial for bone health, especially during the postpartum period when your body may be depleted.

Iron-Rich Foods:

Iron is vital for preventing anemia, which is common postpartum. Red meat, fortified cereals, and legumes are good sources of iron. Pair iron-rich foods with vitamin C sources like citrus fruits to enhance iron absorption.

Hydration and its impact on stretching

Adequate fluid intake is paramount for postpartum recovery. Water is essential for maintaining healthy skin, aiding digestion, and preventing constipation, which is common post-birth. Dehydration is a common issue, especially in warm weather, and it can have serious consequences. To avoid this, follow these guidelines:

- Pre-hydrate by consuming a bottle of water an hour before your stretching.

- Aim to consume at least one 28-ounce bottle of water every hour during your stretching session.

- Don't wait until you feel thirsty to drink. Your body begins to lose fluids before you experience thirst.

- Make it a habit to take a few big sips from your water bottle every 15 minutes during your exercise.

Proper hydration not only aids in the healing process but also helps prevent and manage one of the most common postpartum concerns: skin stretching and the development of stretch marks.

Skin Elasticity:

Hydration is key for skin elasticity, preventing stretch marks. Amply hydrated skin is less prone to stretching damage. Drinking water maintains skin suppleness.

Collagen Production:

Collagen is a key protein for skin structure and strength. the body produces collagen due to adequate hydration, enhancing skin's resilience to stretching.

Healing and Scarring:

Proper hydration aids in the overall healing process, which can affect how well your body repairs any stretch marks or scars resulting from childbirth. Well-hydrated skin is more likely to heal efficiently and potentially reduce the prominence of stretch marks.

Itch and Discomfort:

Dehydrated skin is susceptible to itching and discomfort. It is also prone to stretch marks. Drinking water can ease these symptoms and offer relief.

Chapter 10: Stretches for Emotional Wellbeing

Stretches for Emotional Well-being

The mind-body connection is a powerful one, and maintaining emotional well-being often begins with physical practices that promote relaxation and alleviate tension.

Child's Pose:

In Child's Pose, kneel on the floor, bend forward, extend your arms, and rest your forehead on the ground. This stretch eases lower back and hip tension while promoting mental relaxation.

Cat-Cow Stretch:

Get on your hands and knees, and begin the alternating movement of arching your back, similar to a cat, and curving it, just like a cow's posture. This particular stretch is designed to improve flexibility and relieve tension in your spine. While performing these movements, pay close attention to your breath. Take a deep inhalation during the arch and exhale deeply during the curve.

Seated Forward Bend:

Sit with your legs extended in front of you, then bend forward, reaching for your toes. This stretch lengthens the spine and helps release stress in the neck and shoulders. As you fold, let go of your worries and breathe deeply.

Butterfly Stretch:

Sit with the soles of your feet touching, creating a diamond shape with your legs. Gently press your knees toward the ground. This stretch opens up the hips and groin, and can relieve the physical strain that often accompanies childbirth.

Incorporating these stretches into your daily routine, even if only for a few minutes, can go a long way in promoting emotional well-being. Regular stretching reduces muscle tension, improves circulation, and encourages relaxation, helping you cope with the emotional challenges of the postpartum period.

Coping with Postpartum Emotions

The postpartum period involves significant emotional changes for new parents. Hormonal shifts, sleep deprivation, and the responsibilities of caring for a newborn can evoke a range of emotions, including joy, love, anxiety, and depression. Here are strategies for managing these emotions.

Seek Professional Help:

If your postpartum emotions feel overwhelming or persistent, it's vital to contact a healthcare provider or mental health professional. They can offer guidance, therapy, or medication as needed to assist you through this challenging time.

Open Communication:

Talk to your partner, friends, and family about your emotions. Being open about your feelings can help you feel supported and less isolated. Many new parents have experienced similar emotions and can offer valuable insights and empathy.

Self-Care:

Prioritize self-care. This means taking time for yourself, even if it's just a few minutes a day, to do something that makes you feel relaxed and rejuvenated. This might include a warm bath, reading, meditation, or a short walk.

Acceptance:

Accept that it's okay to have mixed emotions during this period. New parenthood is challenging, and not every moment will be filled with unadulterated joy. Be gentle with yourself and allow space for your emotions to ebb and flow.

Stretches for Stress Relief

Stress is an inevitable part of life, and as a new parent, it can be particularly demanding. Incorporating stress-relieving stretches into your daily routine can help you manage the challenges more effectively.

Neck Rolls:

With a gentle motion, softly rotate your head in a circular fashion, shifting it from one side to the other. This simple stretch has the potential to alleviate tension in the neck and shoulders, common areas where stress tends to build up.

Spinal Twist:

Take a seat with your legs stretched out in front of you. Now, bend one knee and cross it over the opposite leg, while gently twisting your torso to the side. This stretching exercise eases tension in the lower back and encourages a feeling of relaxation.

Legs Up the Wall:

Lie on your back with legs extended upward against a wall. This relaxing posture is known to alleviate stress and aid in relaxation. Keep your eyes closed and concentrate on your breath while maintaining this pose.

Building a Support Network

Creating a support network is essential for maintaining emotional well-being, particularly during the postpartum period. Here are some steps to help build a strong support system.

Connect with Other Parents:

Participate in local parenting circles or virtual discussion platforms, where you can exchange experiences and worries with fellow new parents. These groups offer a source of valuable guidance and emotional assistance.

Lean on Friends and Family:

Don't hesitate to ask friends and family for help when needed. Whether it's a home-cooked meal, a babysitting break, or a listening ear, your loved ones are often more than willing to support you.

Consider Professional Support:

Sometimes, professional guidance is necessary. Reach out to a therapist, counselor, or support group specializing in postpartum issues. They can provide tailored strategies for managing your unique emotional challenges.

Self-Care with a Support System:

Blend self-care with your support system. Encourage a trusted friend or family member to join in self-care endeavors, whether it involves taking a stroll, indulging in a spa day, or just having an open and sincere conversation.

Chapter 11: Beyond the Early Postpartum Period

Staying Active and Flexible as Your Child Grows

Embracing Your New Normal

The postpartum period can be demanding, and as your child grows, you'll likely find it even more challenging to make time for exercise. It's essential to acknowledge that your routine might not resemble your pre-pregnancy workouts. The key is to embrace your new normal and adapt your fitness routine accordingly. Prioritize short, effective workouts that fit into your busy schedule. Aim for flexibility, both in your exercise choices and timing, and don't be too hard on yourself when things don't go as planned.

Incorporating Your Child

As your child grows, incorporating them into your exercise routine can be a fun and effective way to stay active. Baby-wearing during walks or jogs, gentle yoga while your baby plays nearby, or involving your child in low-impact workouts are excellent ways to bond with your little one while getting fit. These activities can also be an opportunity to introduce your child to a healthy lifestyle from an early age.

Joining Mommy-and-Me Fitness Classes

Many fitness centers and community organizations offer Mommy-and-Me fitness classes, which provide a supportive environment for both mothers and children to engage in physical activity. These classes often focus on core strength, flexibility, and cardiovascular fitness while accommodating the presence of young children. It's a wonderful way to socialize with other moms and create a sense of community.

Transitioning to Regular Exercise

Consult with Your Healthcare Provider

Before you transition to regular exercise, it's crucial to consult with your healthcare provider. Your postpartum body may still require special attention, and your healthcare provider can offer valuable guidance. They can help you determine when it's safe to increase the intensity and duration of your workouts and address any concerns you may have about your postpartum recovery.

Gradual Progression

When transitioning to regular exercise, it's essential to progress gradually. Start by incorporating short workouts into your routine, gradually extending the duration and intensity as you regain your strength and stamina. Be attentive to your body's signals and avoid pushing yourself too hard too soon. It's a journey, and patience is key.

Mix It Up

To keep yourself motivated and avoid fatigue, mix up your routines with cardio, strength training, and flexibility. Blend cardio, strength, and flexibility exercises. Cardiovascular workouts, such as jogging, cycling, or swimming, are excellent for overall fitness. Strength training can help you regain muscle tone and metabolic health, while flexibility exercises are essential for maintaining your range of motion and preventing injuries.

Set Realistic Goals

Setting realistic goals is essential when transitioning to regular exercise. These goals should be achievable and tailored to your current fitness level. Whether it's completing a 5K run, doing a certain number of push-ups, or achieving a specific flexibility milestone, setting goals can help you stay motivated and track your progress.

Long-Term Benefits of Postpartum Stretching

Improved Posture and Alignment

Postpartum stretching greatly enhances posture and alignment by addressing musculoskeletal changes resulting from pregnancy and childbirth, reducing discomfort and strain on muscles and joints.

Enhanced Flexibility and Range of Motion

Postpartum stretching routines can enhance your flexibility and range of motion, which is particularly beneficial as your child grows. Being flexible allows you to move more freely during playtime, helps with daily tasks, and makes it easier to keep up with your child as they become more active.

Stress Relief and Mental Well-Being

Caring for a growing child can be overwhelming, and the stress of parenthood can take a toll on your mental well-being. Engaging in postpartum stretching exercises not only relaxes your body but also calms your mind. Practicing deep breathing and mindfulness during your stretching routines can help reduce stress and promote mental clarity.

Injury Prevention

As your child becomes more mobile, there is an increased risk of injuries for mothers who aren't in good physical condition. Postpartum stretching can help prevent injuries by maintaining muscle balance, joint stability, and body awareness. A strong and supple body is less prone to accidents and can recover more quickly if an injury does occur.

Enhanced Postpartum Recovery

Staying consistent with postpartum stretching can expedite your postpartum recovery and help you regain your pre-pregnancy strength. Stretching exercises can target areas that have undergone significant changes during pregnancy and childbirth, such as the abdomen and pelvic floor muscles. This can aid in the healing process and provide a smoother transition to regular exercise.

Conclusion

Your postpartum journey is a unique and transformative experience. This book has equipped you with the knowledge and techniques to aid in your recovery and rejuvenation. Remember that postpartum stretching is not only about physical healing but also about nurturing your emotional and mental well-being. As you embrace the power of postpartum stretches, you are taking a significant step toward a healthier, happier postpartum period and a brighter future with your little one.

Glossary

Postpartum: The period following childbirth.

Stretches: Exercises involving controlled lengthening of muscles.

Posture: The alignment and positioning of the body.

Alignment: The arrangement of body parts in relation to each other.

Discomfort: Mild pain or unease.

Pain: An unpleasant sensation, typically associated with injury or stress.

Stretching Exercises: Physical activities that involve extending the muscles to improve flexibility.

Muscle Strain: Overstretching or injury to a muscle.

Joint Health: The well-being of the connections between bones in the body.

Relaxation: A state of reduced tension and stress.

Core Strength: The power and stability of the body's central muscles.

Pelvic Floor: Muscles, ligaments, and tissues supporting the pelvic organs.

Recovery: The process of healing and returning to a healthy state.

Breath Control: Regulating inhalation and exhalation during exercise.

Flexibility: The ability to bend or stretch without injury.

Lower Back: The region of the back below the ribs and above the hips.

Balance: Stability and equilibrium in the body.

Repetition: The act of doing something multiple times.

Postnatal: Relating to the period after childbirth.

Abdominal Muscles: The muscles in the abdomen, including the rectus abdominis.

Intensity: The degree of force or exertion during an exercise.

Gradual Progression: Incremental development or improvement over time.

Flexor Muscles: Muscles that facilitate bending at joints.

Extension: The straightening of a joint or limb.

Relaxation Techniques: Methods to induce a state of calm and rest.

Hormonal Changes: Alterations in hormone levels in the body.

References

5 exercises and techniques to train for childbirth | Your Pregnancy Matters | UT Southwestern Medical Center. (2016, August 23). Utswmed. https://utswmed.org/medblog/prepare-body-labor-delivery/

Creating A Daily Postpartum Routine. (2022, April 26). The Prima Doula. https://theprimadoula.com/2022/04/25/creating-a-daily-postpartum-routine/?v=1db208cbcff2#:~:text=Don

Cronkleton , E. (2018, January 12). *Tight Shoulders: 12 Stretches for Fast Relief and Tips for Prevention*. Healthline. https://www.healthline.com/health/tight-shoulders

Diastasis Recti (Abdominal Separation): Symptoms & Treatment. (n.d.). Cleveland Clinic. https://my.clevelandclinic.org/health/diseases/22346-diastasis-recti

J Orchard, J., Inge, P., Purdue, R., & W Orchard , J. (2022). *Exercise after pregnancy*. Australian Journal of General Practice. https://www1.racgp.org.au/ajgp/2022/march/exercise-after-pregnancy

Pelvic Floor Exercises for Everyone (Yes, Everyone). (2019, January 24). Healthline. https://www.healthline.com/health/fitness-exercise/pelvic-floor-exercises#benefits-of-strengthening

Postpartum Nutrition Tips to Help Support Recovery. (n.d.). Nutrition news. Retrieved October 28, 2023, from https://www.nutritionnews.abbott/pregnancy-childhood/prenatal-breastfeeding/postpartum-nutrition-tips-to-help-support-recovery/

What are pelvic floor exercises? (2018, June 27). Nhs. https://www.nhs.uk/common-health-questions/lifestyle/what-are-pelvic-floor-exercises/